AVOID CHRONIC DISEASES: STAY OUT OF THE HOSPITAL

A Pocket Reference

By Lena Dobbs-Johnson

The ultimate reference for understanding causes of certain chronic health conditions, protecting your health from chronic disease, and staying out of the hospital

COPYRIGHT INFORMATION

_____

The ideas and considerations detailed in this book are not intended to replace medical advice. All health matters require medical supervision. The author and publisher disclaim any liability arising directly or indirectly from the use of this book.

CONTENTS

INTRODUCTION

The prevalence of obesity and chronic diseases is a huge challenge in this country. A recent report published in October 2012 by the Center for Disease Control and Prevention (CDC) titled *"Fat and getting fatter,"* shows that 35.7% of adults and 16.9% of children ages 2-19 are obese. Many factors contributed to the rapid decline in health since the industrial revolution. One of the biggest factors is the development of the "fast foods industry." Most of what is produced in fast foods contains high fat and high sugar, fueling obesity and chronic diseases. The fast food industry has grown by leaps and bounds over the past decades. Thanks to creative marketing efforts geared especially to younger people, the fast food evolution is now like an unstoppable locomotive.

In addition to the fast food industry, and more recently, there is a proliferation of food and cooking shows on many TV networks. Many of these shows demonstrate unhealthy cooking, further contributing to obesity and heart disease. I was in a spa getting a pedicure and watched a food show on TV. What I saw was alarming to me and everyone in the shop who saw this gasped. The cook demonstrating the recipe fried a pack of bacon on the stove and placed the bacon strips aside to drain when they were finished. The bacon generated one-third cup of oil which she used added to a mixture of milk, eggs, butter, corn, flour, some seasonings and crumbled bacon then placed it in the oven to bake. Another food show on TV included contestants pigging out on five pounds of burger or 24 hot dogs in one sitting. These are some of the factors contributing to an obesity crises and chronic health challenges in the United States. Other factors include sedentary lifestyles, food desserts, fad diets, lack of, and or confusing information about healthy eating, weight loss and causes of disease.

Regardless of the causes, the evidence is clear. The poor health of a majority of Americans is costing individuals heavily in terms of pain, suffering, doctor and medication bills and costing the government billions of dollars each year.

Unfortunately, there is little evidence that this situation is changing as fast as we would like to see it change. This situation will require multiple efforts to help create change. The Affordable Care Act that became law in 2014 has some meaningful components including a focus on preventive care and health promotion. But that too will take time. Other factors and groups that are helping include; lawmakers passing meaningful regulations to minimize harmful ingredients in foods and requiring better labeling so that people know what is in the food that they are consuming; continuing actions of lobbying groups that fight for good nutrition, employers developing incentives to promote healthy lifestyles among employees, and more meaningful and responsible food shows on cable networks. Also, a wellness focused rather than disease or sickness focused health care industry will help produce positive changes.

But most importantly, in addition to all of the above, we must make sure that consumers have the information to make intelligent decisions. Here again, how does the consumer get the best information when they are trying to educate themselves on safe food products, and what foods are part of a healthy and balanced diet? The Internet is full of information. At the click of a button you can find information on any topic. Some of this information is useful and others are confusing and less helpful. Numerous health food and herbal products are on the market and they too make many claims about the ability of their products to cure or improve certain conditions. Also, many news networks will report research findings as part of a telecast but these lack details.

With such plethora of information what are consumers supposed to do? Rely on the advice of their health care practitioner who they barely see once each year if that much? Furthermore, some doctors do not take calls from patients to answer basic questions. The bottom-line is that consumers need to take personal responsibility for their health and wellbeing.

The purpose of this book is to give everyday consumers who want to make important health changes some basic road maps to help make those changes. The book is not a medical book but one that focuses on lifestyle changes. It is written in an easy to understand language. Consumers may go directly to the section that applies to them or to anyone else they want to help. It is small enough to carry and use as a pocket reference.

CHAPTER 1 - READING FOOD LABELS

Almost all of us purchase packaged foods at one time or another either because the food is seasonal, or because we need to find something to eat very quickly. Whatever the reason, we need to know how to select food that will not compromise our health, and this is where understanding how to read food labels comes in.

Determining what information is on a food label and how to decipher it may be intimidating to some people. The next section will provide a step-by-step guide to help you.

The good news is that food labels are regulated in the United States. Certain sections on all labels are standard and regulated by the government. Very soon, the government will be mandating changes to food labels to make it easier for consumers to understand. The total calories and servings per container information will most likely be in very bold font.

Here is a sample of a typical food label with additional explanations:

NUTRITION LABEL

Shows all mandatory requirements found on all food labels except meat and poultry.

(1) START HERE

Nutrition Facts

Serving Size 1 Cookie (19g)
Servings Per Container 10

Understand how many servings are in the container. This is one of the areas that the government has proposed changing to

Amount Per Serving

(2) CHECK CALORIES

Calories 90   Calories from Fat 30 — Proposed to be bigger and bolder.

	% Daily Value*
Total Fat 3.5g	**5%**
Saturated Fat 1g	**5%**
Trans Fat 0g	
Cholesterol 5mg	**2%**
Sodium 25mg	**1%**
Total Carbohydrate 13g	**4%**
Dietary Fiber 1g	**4%**
Sugars 9g	
Protein 1g	

(3) LIMIT THESE NUTRIENTS

— Saturated fat. Bad, try to limit.

— Trans fat also called partially hydrogenated oil. Bad, avoid.

(Monounsaturated and poly-unsaturated fat - Good fats)

— Look for foods with higher fiber and lower sugar.

(4) GET ENOUGH OF THESE NUTRIENTS

Vitamin A 2%	•	Vitamin C 0%
Calcium 2%	•	Iron 2%

New minerals like vitamin D and potassium will be added in this section.

(5) FOOTNOTE

*Percent Daily Values are based on a 2,000 calorie diet. Your daily values may be higher or lower depending on your calorie needs:

	Calories:	2,000	2,500
Total Fat	Less than	65g	80g
Saturated Fat	Less than	20g	25g
Cholesterol	Less than	300mg	300mg
Sodium	Less than	2,400mg	2,400mg
Total Carbohydrate		300g	375g
Dietary Fiber		25g	30g

Calories per gram:
Fat 9 • Carbohydrate 4 • Protein 4

(6) INGREDIENTS

INGREDIENTS: SUGAR, ENRICHED FLOUR (WHEAT FLOUR, MALTED BARLEY FLOUR, NIACIN, IRON, THIAMINE MONONITRATE, RIBOFLAVIN, FOLIC ACID), ALMONDS BUTTER (CREAM), NATURAL FLAVORS, BROWN RICE SYRUP, SALT, CINNAMON.

The ingredient section is not mandated, but is a very important area to read. Ingredients are listed in order from the highest amount in the product to the least.

At the bottom of the label is allergen information that is also very important. Somewhere on the label is the manufacturer's contact information in case of questions or recalls.

(7) ALLERGEN WARNING

Contains Wheat, Almonds, Milk.

SUMMARY CONSIDERATIONS

•   Pay attention to serving sizes because a container may have several servings.

•   Look for trans fats and saturated fats. These are the bad fats.

•   Look for hydrogenated and partially hydrogenated oils.

These are bad.

- High sugar under the carbohydrate total indicates low quality carbohydrates.

- Look for food dyes and flavor enhancers like MSG (also called autolyzed yeast.)

- Pay attention to "OSE." Most products containing this include some form of sugar-like sucrose, fructose, high fructose corn syrup, etc.

Read the ingredient section very carefully because it tells what is in the food. There may be allergen information that you need to be aware of. Also, pay attention to food dyes and ingredient names that are hard to pronounce.

CHAPTER 2 - UNDERSTANDING GOOD AND BAD CARBOHYDRATES

Carbohydrates are specific types of food that are needed to provide fuel to the brain. When we eat carbohydrate food, it is broken down into glucose to provide that fuel. Carbohydrates are classified as either complex or simple according to their effect on the body.

Complex carbohydrates (good) take longer to break down and digest so they do not cause a rapid increase in blood sugar levels. Because of this, complex carbohydrates are lower on the glycemic index scale.

Simple carbohydrates (bad) are high on the glycemic index scale, meaning that they break down very quickly and can raise the blood sugar level rapidly. Excesses of the simple carbohydrates can cause weight gain and with it the corresponding problems of obesity, heart disease, and diabetes. Additionally, according to the Harvard Medical, "bad carbohydrates can affect your triglycerides and HDL cholesterol levels."

So, now that you know that there are good and bad carbohydrates, you may be asking what are they? The next page identifies both types of carbohydrates, and shows sources of both.

TWO TYPES OF CARBOHYDRATES	
"Good" Carbohydrates are also called **Complex Carbohydrates.** They are full of nutrients and are excellent brain food.	"Bad" Carbohydrates are also called **Simple Carbohydrates.** These have no nutrients and are often called empty calories. Eliminate or limit these for a healthy diet.
Sources/Examples • Yams • Beans • Whole grains, legumes • Brown rice • Millet, barley • Bran • Vegetables including green, leafy vegetables, cabbage, cauliflower, broccoli, okra, spinach, and mushrooms	Sources/Examples • Pasta • Crackers • Cake • White rice • Cereals • Sugar, soda • Honey

SUMMARY

- Choose complex carbohydrates over simple ones when planning your meals.

- When looking at the carbohydrate count on food labels, those with higher amounts of sugar are usually the refined ones, so stay away from them

CHAPTER 3 - PROTEIN

Protein is essential for life. The main role of protein is for growth and tissue repair. When protein foods are eaten they are broken down into amino acids. Amino acids build and repair cells, strengthen the immune system, promote healthy skin and hair, and help to provide hormones and enzymes needed for digestion. There are about 22 amino acids in the body. Some of them are called non-essential because the body makes them. However, there are nine amino acids that are called essential, meaning that they have to come from the food we eat.

Although proteins from animal, poultry, eggs, and fish sources have all the essential amino acids the body needs, it is best to consume protein from a variety of sources.

We just learned that there are non-essential and essential proteins. Now let's review them and list some sources.

TWO TYPES OF PROTEIN	
ESSENTIAL PROTEINS This type of protein has all nine essential amino acids and has to be obtained from the foods we consume.	NON-ESSENTIAL PROTEINS This type of protein does not have all nine essential amino acids and are easily made in the body.
Sources/Examples • Animal products • Poultry • Milk and cheese products • Eggs • Fish	Sources/Examples • Beans • Legumes • Grains • Seeds • Nuts

CHAPTER 4 - GOOD AND BAD FATS

Fat is needed in the body. However, just like carbohydrates, not all fats are created equal. Some fats are absolutely necessary and good for the body; others are dangerous. Here is a good way to distinguish good and bad fats, as well as, where to look for them.

Good fats are needed in a healthy diet to assist with metabolic processes. They also help to build and repair cell membranes in the brain and heart, and most importantly, support the immune system. These good fats also help to reduce inflammation.

Dangerous fats stifle the immune system and predispose a person to cancer and other degenerative diseases. They raise triglyceride and bad cholesterol levels, increasing the risk of heart disease, stroke, and death. Bad fats stay in the bloodstream for long periods of time because they are difficult to break down.

Now that we know that there are good and bad fats let's look at sources of both. My goal is to keep this as simple as possible so that you will use the information to improve your health.

See chart on the next page.

TYPES OF FATS

GOOD FATS

There are two main types of good fats. They are:

1. Monounsaturated fats

    Main sources are avocados, olives, canola oil, sesame, olive oil.

2. Polyunsaturated (healthiest)

    (a) Omega-3 fatty acids
    Found in oily fish like sardines, herring, wild salmon, mackerel, anchovies, fortified omega eggs, and nuts like hazelnuts, pecans, cashews, brazil nuts.

    (b) Omega-6 fatty acids
    Corn oil, cotton-seed oil, safflower oil, sunflower oil, soybeans, and walnuts.

BAD FATS

There are two main types of bad fats. They are:

1. Saturated fats

    Main sources are animal products, cheese, butter, lard, ice cream, palm oil, cream cheese, animal shortening, and processed fatty meats like pepperoni, sausages, hot dogs, and bacon.

2. Trans fats AKA partially hydrogenated fats

    (a) Trans-fat is manmade. Hydrogen is pumped through vegetable oil and the liquid then turns solid.

    (b) Trans-fats are also found in doughnuts, cakes, fried foods, processed meats, packaged goods, muffins, pizza, and candy bars. Trans fats prolong the shelf life of many of these products.

Tips for a healthy lifestyle

- Eat avocados on salads
- Use olive oil in salad dressing
- Eat a variety of fish
- Eat nuts and olives as described above *
- Supplement with fish oil if not contraindicated; for example if you are taking blood thinning medication, avoid the supplement.
- Cooking oils with a good ratio of saturated, monounsaturated, and polyunsaturated fat include canola, grape seed, and sunflower oils.

Check allergen information on nuts

Tips to avoid dangerous fats

- When shopping read labels carefully. If partially hydrogenated oil is listed stay away from it. Again, partially hydrogenated fats are the same as trans fats.
- Avoid commercially baked goods listed above.
- Bake, broil, steam, and eat lean cuts of meat if you are a meat eater.
- Do not use olive oil to fry. When it is heated above its smoke point it breaks down and becomes bad.

CHAPTER 5 - UNDERSTANDING CHOLESTEROL

Today millions of Americans are taking some form of cholesterol lowering drug. Although cholesterol discussion is commonplace in our culture, I suspect that many people do not know the basics of cholesterol; what it is, why they should be concerned if their cholesterol is high, and what doctor's look for on cholesterol tests. Hopefully by reading these pages you will get answers to these questions.

Cholesterol is a fatty substance found in everyone's body. There are two main sources of cholesterol. Serum cholesterol is normally made by the body and accounts for about 80 percent of cholesterol. Dietary cholesterol comes from the food we eat — mainly animal protein — and accounts for about 20 percent.

The main components of cholesterol are total cholesterol that is made up of high density lipoprotein (HDL) and low density lipoprotein (LDL). A third form of fat called triglyceride is also considered.

Here are the different components explained in more detail. The ranges are as of 2012 and can change slightly depending on the laboratory and new information from medical associations.

When the doctor orders a cholesterol test, also called a lipid panel, the LDL and HDL ranges, as well as total cholesterol are all done. Cholesterol/HDL ratio, and triglyceride levels are also included.

See the following chart:

TYPES OF CHOLESTEROL

HDL (Good)	LDL (Bad)	Triglycerides
High density lipoprotein (HDL) is the good part of cholesterol. According to the Harvard Medical School Guide to Lowering Your Cholesterol, "HDL acts like a vacuum cleaner, sucking up extra cholesterol from cells and tissues and takes it back to the liver which takes the cholesterol out of the particles and either uses it to make bile or recycles it."[1] Because of this factor, higher HDL helps to lower cholesterol levels.	Low density Lipoprotein (LDL) is the bad part of cholesterol. LDL predisposes the blood to clot. LDL is the form of cholesterol that deposits plaque in the arteries that can eventually cause blockage and heart attacks. This is why the higher the LDL, the more dangerous the cholesterol.	In addition to looking at HDL, LDL, and cholesterol ratios, doctors typically look at triglyceride levels. Triglycerides are stored fats in the body. An excess of saturated fats and trans fats cause high triglyceride levels. (See the chapter on fats) Triglycerides are dangerous because they make the blood thicker, thereby more likely to form clots.
Normal range: > 39 mg/dL	Normal range: <100<mg/dL	Normal range: < 150mg/dL

Here is how to calculate the cholesterol /HDL ratio:

If your total cholesterol is.......210

And if your HDL is 50

Then your Cholesterol/HDL ratio is 210/50 = 4.2

Ideal ratio is now 0-3.6 for most labs

To recap, health care practitioners look at:

• Total cholesterol

• LDL

• HDL

• Total Cholesterol/HDL ratio

• LDL/HDL ratio

• Triglycerides

At this point you may be wondering how triglycerides fit in the picture? A high triglyceride level, with high LDL (bad) cholesterol is normally a dangerous combination. That is why triglyceride levels are included in the cholesterol /lipid panel.

CONSIDERATIONS TO HELP FIGHT HIGH CHOLESTEROL/TRIGLYCERIDE PROBLEM

If your cholesterol is high, working with your health care practitioner is important. However, it is your health, so take responsibility to make the changes necessary to improve it. Furthermore, you live with yourself every day, and most people do not see a health care practitioner more than once each year if that often.

So, consider making some basic lifestyle changes:

CONSIDER THESE	AVOID THESE
Dietary considerations • Eat well balanced meals with lots of fruits and vegetables. • Increase intake of monounsaturated and polyunsaturated fats, omega-3 oily fish, olives, olive oil, avocados, nuts, canola oil, and sunflower seeds. • High levels of polyunsaturated fats help to lower triglycerides and can be found in walnuts, flaxseed, and safflower oil. • Fiber. Increase fiber intake, especially soluble fiber from sources like oat-bran, apples, and citrus. Green, leafy vegetables have an abundance of fiber. Beans, legumes, and prunes also have high fiber that may help to lower cholesterol. • All forms of nuts are good for lowering cholesterol, but do not overdo it because they are also high in calories. **Exercise** Exercise has tremendous health benefits, so consider adding some form of exercise to your daily routine. Choose exercises that fit into your lifestyle and health status. **Lose Weight** If you are overweight, try to lose weight and get your BMI to the normal range. You will see a reduction in your total cholesterol even with moderate weight loss.	• Trans fats. These are enemies to a healthy heart. They are found in most of your processed factory foods like potato chips and French fries. • Saturated fats found in animal products, cheese, ice cream, processed meats. • Alcohol and sugar. • If you smoke, reduce or eliminate smoking. • Sedentary lifestyle.

CHAPTER 6 - SUGAR

Today, sugar is a staple in the majority of desserts and most processed foods. Sugar can be extremely detrimental to your health and should be better known as the sweet deception. All sugar is high on the glycemic index, meaning it goes through the bloodstream very rapidly causing a surge in glucose. Unstable blood glucose is linked to weight gain. Furthermore, sugar causes binges and cravings. When you fill up on sugar, you are hungry a few hours later because you have just eaten empty calories.

A variety of studies have described the dangers associated with sugar. One cancer researcher, Wayne Martin, notes that, "when someone eats sugar, the body produces insulin, and insulin can promote breast cancer just as estrogen does." He also noted that sugar reduces the effectiveness of the immune system. This reduced effectiveness can last up to five hours.[2]

Sugar is addictive, and in addition to cravings, it causes a host of other bad conditions. Let's review the effects of excess sugar below.

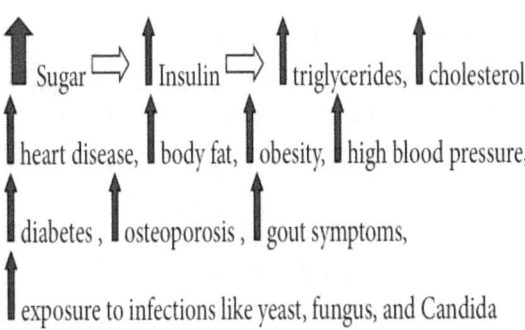

SUGAR FREE/SUGARLESS

Sometimes people trying to avoid sugar buy sugar free or sugarless products. Sugar free and sugarless on a label means the product does not have sucrose or some of the other sweeteners we know, but may still contain one or more of the sugar alcohols like xylitol, mannitol, sorbital, or other artificial sweeteners like aspartame. Sugar alcohols are not bad. Although they have the same number of calories as regular sugar, they are not absorbed from the small intestines, so they do not affect blood sugar levels and are safer for diabetics to use. Aspartame, on the other hand, is an artificial sweetener that may be linked to health issues.[3]

THE HONEY MYTH

Many people assume that it is better to use honey rather than sugar and may proudly declare, "I do not use sugar, I use honey." The truth is that honey is similar to table sugar. Table sugar has pure sucrose, while honey has fructose, glucose, and sucrose. If you are still not convinced, consider this:

• 1 teaspoon of table sugar has 46 calories

• 1 teaspoon of honey has 64 calories

• Furthermore, most honey is now processed and is high on the glycemic index, and raises blood sugar quickly.

HOW TO RECOGNIZE SUGAR IN PRODUCTS

Sugar is known by many names so here is a guide to help you recognize hidden sugar in your products. Look for:

1.   Dextrose - Also called glucose and is chemically produced from cornstarch

2.   Corn syrup - From cornstarch treated with enzymes to produce sucrose, fructose, and glucose

3.   Fructose - Natural fruit sugar

4.   Glucose - See dextrose. From fruits, honey, and vegetables

5.   Honey - Produced by bees from the nectar of flowers. Has fructose, glucose, and sucrose

6.   Lactose - Sugar in milk and dairy products

7.   Maltose/malt sugar - Found in germinating seeds

8.   Sugar alcohols - Includes sorbitol, xylitol, mannitol

9.   Maple syrup - From maple tree sap

10.   Molasses - End product of sucrose extraction from sugar cane

11.   Sucrose - From sugar cane or sugar beets (granulated raw, turbinado, brown) sugar, invert sugar[4]

A BETTER SUBSTITUTE

If you are trying to reduce the use of sugar, think about substituting the sugar or honey with:

1.   Sugar alcohols - xylitol, sorbitol, and mannitol. These are not absorbed from the small intestines and can be safely used by diabetics.

2.   Sweet leaf stevia. There are some stevia products on the shelves that are processed. Please read labels and avoid these.

3.   Honey. If you must use honey consider raw, natural manuka honey.

4.   The jury is still out on the other sugar substitutes like aspartame, saccharin, and Sweet N'Low. I personally avoid these.

CHAPTER 7 - THE COLON AND ROLE OF FIBER

The colon is one of the three parts of the large intestines. The three parts are the cecum, colon, and rectum. The colon has some important functions:

• It is the storehouse for the end products of the food we eat before it is passed out.

• It is the home for millions of friendly bacteria that manufacture enzymes to break down the plant fiber that we consume.

• The flora in this area also makes vitamin K that is needed for the clotting of blood.

• Water from the food we eat and digest is pulled out in colon to leave a more solid content that is stored until it is ready to be eliminated as a bowel movement.

The foods we eat affect the function of the colon in either good or bad ways. For example, processed fatty meats, deep fried foods, excess sugar, and a low fiber diet adversely affect the colon and cause constipation and irregular bowel moments. It is important to evacuate dead, unwanted products from the colon on a regular basis. According to Linda Berry, "Even with one bowel movement per day you still have at least three meal's worth of waste sitting in your colon most of the time." On the other hand when we eat a diet of fruits and complex carbohydrates as well as fiber it affects the colon in good ways in that it helps with proper elimination as well as helps prevent disease formation like colon cancer.[5]

When food stays in the colon for an extended period, it has more time to rot and can cause brain fog, body odor, headache, fatigue, and possibly colon cancer.

FIBER

One of the best ingredients for a healthy colon is fiber. The standard American diet is deficient in fiber. Many people are unaware of the value of fiber or even understand its role. Simply stated, fiber is the roughage in food.

It will help you achieve your weight loss goal and a lot more. Fiber is a friend to overall health and wellness. Let's review some of the many health benefits that can be attributed to fiber.

• Keeping a person feeling full, thereby controlling hunger and preventing overeating.

• Stabilizing blood sugar so the demand for insulin is reduced. This has a positive effect on controlling rapid increases and decreases in blood sugar that could eventually cause health problems.

• Functioning like a broom to sweep toxins from the intestinal walls before they stagnate and cause disease. There are some schools of thought that believe extra fiber in the diet will reduce the incidence of colon cancer.

• Reducing constipation which may also be a factor in reducing colon cancer. Irritable bowel syndrome is improved by the addition of extra fiber in the diet.

• Reducing bad cholesterol (LDL), which helps to reduce total cholesterol and heart disease.

• Fiber binds toxic substances in the colon so they are not absorbed to cause harm to the body.

TYPES OF FIBER

There are two types of fiber: soluble and insoluble. Soluble fiber becomes gel-like when mixed with water, e.g. pectin and mucilage. Insoluble fiber passes through the digestive tract without being digested.

See the diagram.

Soluble Fiber	Insoluble Fiber
Gel-like and purports to lower cholesterol	Insoluble...unchanged, soft, bulky, absorbs water and has no effect on cholesterol
SOURCES • Oat bran, rice bran, barley, oatmeal • Lentils • Flax • Brussels sprouts, broccoli, cabbage • Sweet potatoes • Apples, strawberries, peaches • Prunes and raisins Note: Prunes are high in calories so watch the serving size.	SOURCES • Navy beans • Black beans • Kidney beans • Chick peas • Lima beans • Black-eyed peas • Apples

CONSIDERATIONS FOR A HEALTHY COLON

•	A diet high in fiber, complex carbohydrates, fruits, and vegetables has been shown to help maintain regular bowel movements and a healthy colon.

•	Avoid processed and fried foods that tend to cause constipation.

•	Drink plenty of water and keep the body hydrated.

•	Regular detoxification of the body is an excellent way to help ensure a healthy colon.

•	Some people add probiotics to their daily regimen. This helps to feed the friendly bacteria in the colon and assist with overall colon health.

CHAPTER 8 - BODY MASS INDEX (BMI)

The debate about how much a person should weigh, based on their height, facilitated the development of the body mass index, which is a fairly accurate way of establishing what a person's weight should be based on their height. The body mass index is a ratio of weight to height. The BMI is based on the metric system. Pounds and inches are usually converted to kilograms and meters. However, for people unfamiliar with the metric system, the BMI can be calculated using pounds and inches. This methodology is easy to calculate and is now widely used in health and wellness programs.

The ranges established for BMI are listed below:

Level	BMI Range	Indication
1	< 18.5	Underweight
2	18.6-24.9	Normal
3	25-29.9	Overweight
4	30-39.9	Obese
5	Over 40	Extremely obese

The higher the BMI, the more obese the person is, and the higher the risk of diabetes and cardiovascular diseases. The BMI is a simple tool that can be used to gauge whether a person is obese.

CALCULATING YOUR BMI

How do you determine your BMI without looking to

health professionals? There are two basic methods. We will use Sammy's weight and height to show how both formulas work:

Conversion:	Sammy:	Weight 176 lbs.
1 lb. = 2.2 kilos		Height 6' 0"
1 inch = 2.54 cm		
1 inch = .0254 meter		

How to calculate BMI when using Pounds	How to calculate BMI when using Metric system
<u>Weight in pounds</u> (Height² in.) x 703	<u>Weight in kilos</u> (Height cm. x height cm.)

<u>176</u>
    (72 x 72)   x 703 =
24
	<u>80</u>
	    (183 x 183) =
	24

FOR CONSIDERATION

• Calculate your own BMI and know what your numbers represent.

• If your BMI is above the normal range, lose weight and embark on a healthy lifestyle changes including proper eating, exercise, rest, and detoxification.

• Follow-up with your health care professional on a regular basis.

CHAPTER 9 - GLYCEMIC INDEX

Many people who are trying to eat properly or lose weight have been warned about avoiding foods with a high glycemic index. Diabetics have also been warned about these foods. However, many people do not know what the index is or why high glycemic index foods are dangerous, so let us try to provide some guidance.

The glycemic index is a formula used to determine how quickly foods containing carbohydrates are broken down to glucose and subsequently how fast the blood sugar level is raised. Rapid rises in blood sugar trigger an excessive release of insulin to help get rid of the sugar. When we eat, our blood sugar naturally rises, but blood sugar levels that rise and fall excessively contribute to many health problems as noted in the chapter on insulin resistance.

The glycemic index applies only to carbohydrates. Protein and fats are not considered on this scale. There is a range on the glycemic index from 0-100. Zero is considered low and 100 is high. Any carbohydrate that raises blood sugar quickly after consumption is considered to be high on the glycemic index. High glycemic foods are mainly processed foods; however, there are some non-processed foods that are high on the glycemic index. See the following chart:

GLYCEMIC INDEX SCALE

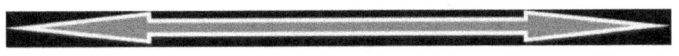

LOW	MODERATE	HIGH
0% - 55 %	56 - 69%	70% - 100%

CHART OF SOME GLYCEMIC INDEX FOODS

LOW	MODERATE	HIGH
Complex carbohydrates like brown rice, whole grains Vegetables: beans, broccoli, cauliflower Fruits: apples, peaches, pears	Beans Brown rice Bananas	Processed foods All forms of sugar Cakes, cookies Bagels, waffles, pancakes Honey Jams and jelly White rice, white flour Fruit juice

CONSIDERATIONS

• Try to avoid high glycemic foods, if possible. You may not be able to do so consistently, but consciously paying attention to these foods will produce many health benefits. For example, it could prevent development of Type 2 diabetes, high cholesterol/triglycerides, and high blood pressure.

• Some health professionals believe that rapid increases in blood sugar levels can be avoided by eating protein along with high glycemic foods. For example, eating almond butter or cheese with crackers.

CHAPTER 10 - DIETING AND WEIGHT LOSS FACTS

AND FADS

Every day, millions of Americans are on a diet and many are repeat dieters. In addition, each year Americans spend over $50 billion on diet products and diet aids. Despite these stunning statistics, a 2012 study by the Center for Disease Control (CDC), labeled *"Fat and Getting Fatter,"* revealed that 35.7 percent of adults and 16.9 percent of children are overweight.

Every day people are bombarded with information about weight loss from TV, the Internet, social media, books, magazines, web ads, and a lot more. Most of these offer quick fixes. The information is sometimes confusing and contradictory, but people gravitate to these quick fixes, looking for the magic bullet only to find out later that there isn't one.

One of the main reasons diets do not work is because they are based on the wrong philosophy, as noted by Mark MacDonald in *Body Confidence*.[6] These diets are products of what is called yo-yo dieting that is based on calorie restriction, starvation, cravings, lack, quick fixes, magic bullets, and Band-Aids. Calorie restriction causes a person to temporarily lose some weight, but it also causes lean muscle loss. Once lean muscle is lost, the metabolism slows down; making it harder to lose fat. As noted by Dr. Lance Levy, "When we lose lean body tissue, however, we are losing the very tissue that is responsible for sustaining our metabolic rate. A cycle of weight gain/weight loss/weight gain causes a progressively higher body fat content and lower muscle content."[7]

Some people will lose weight rapidly and feel good, only to see their weight rise quickly back to their previous weight and more. According to Wendy Murphy, in a *USA Today* health report published in September 2012, 44 percent returned to their original weigh, and 27 percent gained more than they lost after a popular weight loss program. Only 12 percent kept the weight off with ease.[8]

A LIFESTYLE CHANGE MODEL

MORE OF THESE	AVOID THESE
FOOD	FOOD
Many studies have shown that the following habits will contribute to a healthy lifestyle and weight loss.	The main food items that jeopardize a healthy lifestyle and should be minimized are:
• Eat complex carbohydrates like whole grains, brown rice, baked sweet potatoes, and vegetables. • If you eat meat, eat lean cuts of meat and fish. • Let fiber be your friend. Fiber keeps you full so you do not overeat. It also helps to stabilize the blood sugar. Soluble fiber also helps lower cholesterol. • Eat a variety of green, raw vegetables and fruits on a regular basis. • consume at least six glasses of water each day. If you are finding it hard to drink water consider adding mint leaves, lemon slices, cucumber slices, or other fruits to flavor and sip rather than drink throughout the day.	• Sugar of all kinds, including honey. All sugar is high glycemic, meaning it goes through the bloodstream very rapidly, causing a surge in glucose. Unstable blood glucose is linked to weight gain. Furthermore, sugar causes binges and cravings. Once you fill up on sugar, a few hours later you are hungry again and want to eat because there are empty calories in sugar. Sugar can be extremely detrimental to your health according to many research studies. • Processed foods and refined carbohydrates like white rice, pasta, most cereal— especially quick-fix microwave cereals, cake, cookies, and bread. They are enemies to a stable weight. • Trans fats and saturated fats found mainly in fried foods and packaged goods. • Alcohol. One ounce of alcohol has more calories than one gram of carbohydrates. • Fruit juices. They are high on the glycemic index and increase blood sugar levels quickly. • Dairy and soy. These help to sabotage weight loss. Dairy causes mucus and inflammation.
EXERCISE Engage in some moderate exercise. Even walking or swimming helps the heart and overall health.	
SLEEP Get adequate sleep to help the body's cells regenerate. Lack of sleep retards weight loss progress and may cause the release of the fat storing hormone.	OTHER ITEMS TO BE AVOIDED
EXTRAS • Nip cravings in the bud. If you are still hungry after eating it means that you have not eaten the right ratio of protein, carbohydrate, and fats. It also may mean that you have eaten high glycemic foods that get broken down too quickly into glucose. • Detox your body regularly. There are many products on the market that can be used. Be kind to your body and flush out the junk at least quarterly, with the changing seasons • When eating out, avoid gravies, pasta, and foods mentioned on right hand side of this chart.	• Any weight loss plan that contains the word diet. • Quick weight loss plans using pills, herbs, calorie restriction, and starvation. • Weight loss plans that do not include lifestyle changes.

CHAPTER 11 - METABOLIC SYNDROME

You may have heard medical practitioners refer to the term metabolic syndrome and wonder what they are talking about. Metabolic syndrome is medical terminology used to describe a group of risk factors that may lead to life threatening diseases. A person with metabolic syndrome has at least three or more of the following risk conditions:

1.   High blood pressure >130/85mg/Hg

2.   High triglycerides >150 mg/dL

3.   Low HDL cholesterol <40 mg/dL

4.   Large waist >35" female and >40" male

5.   Fasting blood sugar >110mg/dL[9]

Obviously, one of these risk factors alone is a problem, but when combined with two or three more, the risk is increased.

YOUR OPTIONS WITH METABOLIC SYNDROME

If you are told that you have metabolic syndrome it is time to get very serious about working on your health. In addition to working with your doctor there are things that you can do to improve the condition. There are specific chapters in this book dealing with high blood pressure, high cholesterol, diabetes, and obesity. Review those chapters. This section is just a recap of those chapters.

a.   High cholesterol - Cholesterol is a fatty substance that floats in the bloodstream in the body. There are two sources of cholesterol in the body: 1) cholesterol that is naturally made by the body; and, 2) cholesterol from food, mainly animal protein. See chapter on cholesterol.

b.   High blood pressure - High blood pressure also called hypertension (blood pressure reading of >150/90 mg/Hg) affects millions of Americans each year. This is a chronic condition that can lead to a stroke, so it is important to check the blood pressure regularly. Work with your doctor to control high blood pressure. In addition, here are few suggestions that will help maintain a healthy blood pressure:

•   Reduce processed meat like bacon, hot dogs, sausages, and red meat.

•   Reduce fried foods and foods containing hydrogenated fats like those found in baked goods and potato chips.

•   Reduce intake of salt in the diet. Read labels to make sure there is no extra salt in canned goods.

•   It is best to bake, steam, or broil foods.

•   Eat plenty of fresh fruits and vegetables.

•   Get moderate exercise each day and drink plenty of water.

•   Reduce stress levels by meditating, listening to music, or by other methods you find helpful.

c.   Diabetes - Diabetes refers to high levels of sugar circulating in the blood stream. The most common type of diabetes and the one we will discuss here is Type 2. This is the non-insulin dependent diabetes. One of the main causes of Type 2 diabetes is obesity. Therefore, one of the easiest ways to control the disease is to lose weight. Additionally, avoid processed foods that have a high glycemic index— meaning that they get broken down quickly and enter the blood stream where they cause a rapid increase in blood sugar. So, avoid high glycemic foods like watermelon, white rice, bread, sugar, processed cereals, bagels, and baked goods.

Taking personal responsibility for lifestyle changes, paying attention to what we eat, and increasing our level of physical activity are excellent tools to manage diabetes.

INSULIN RESISTANCE AND PRE-DIABETES

Insulin resistance occurs when excess glucose builds up in the blood instead of being absorbed by the cells. This happens because the cells are not responding as they should to insulin. To help explain this process further, let us look at the interaction of glucose and insulin:

• When we eat carbohydrates, glucose levels surge. To counteract this, the pancreas releases insulin to absorb the excess glucose and carry it into the cells where it can be used as energy.

• Routinely abusing our bodies by eating excess refined carbohydrates and high glycemic foods will constantly place a surge of glucose in the blood. When this happens and insulin tries to escort sugar into the cells, the cells are too full. The body, therefore tries to get the sugar out of the bloodstream the best way it can either by 1) storing it as fat around the belly, 2) contributing to onset of diabetes and/or, 3) increasing cholesterol levels.

WHAT CAUSES INSULIN RESISTANCE?

Many studies have reported that these factors may have a role in contributing to insulin resistance.

• Constant abuse of the body, by eating high glycemic food, makes it harder and harder for the pancreas to keep producing enough insulin to meet the body's glucose demands.

• Excess weight that helps to trigger excess insulin.

• Excess belly fat that triggers excess insulin.

• A sedentary lifestyle tends to increase weight that triggers excess insulin.

PRE-DIABETES

Pre-diabetes is a condition that occurs when the lab numbers for blood sugar levels are close, but not quite at the diabetic level. Pre-diabetes is a warning that unless treatment or lifestyle changes occur, the condition will eventually lead to full diabetes.

There are at least three tests that practitioners look at when making a diagnosis of pre-diabetes:

	TEST	NORMAL RANGE
1.	Hemoglobin (HbA1c). This test measures glucose levels over a three month period of time. In pre-diabetes the hemoglobin A1C is higher than normal, but not at the diabetes level.	5.7% - 6.4%
2.	Fasting glucose.	100 -125mg/dL
3.	Glucose tolerance test (IGTT) This test measures glucose levels after no consumption of glucose for eight hours and again, two hours after ingesting a sweet drink.	140mg/dL

CONSIDERATIONS TO REDUCE PROGRESSION AND RISK

Once you know your numbers for these tests, if you are in the borderline range there are changes that you can make to improve the numbers. Lifestyle changes are the most important consideration mentioned in almost all health literature. Some of these changes include:

1.   Eating regularly to allow insulin ranges to be stable. Skipping meals is unhealthy for glucose stabilization.

2.   Losing weight. If you are overweight, lose weight and get your body mass index (BMI) to within normal levels. As you do

this, avoid yo-yo dieting products and aids.

3.   Modifying what you eat by evaluating what you currently eat and gradually replacing unhealthy choices with good choices. Healthy meals include low glycemic, high fiber foods, and lots of fruits and vegetables.

4.   Paying attention to your digestion and seeing how long it takes to digest your food. Many people are gluten intolerant and do not know that they have the allergy. Typically, these people tend to have a hard time losing weight. If you are concerned about gluten intolerance you can get tested.

5.   Exercising on a regular basis and avoiding a sedentary lifestyle.

6.   Reducing stress and getting adequate sleep. Both of these contribute to a healthy lifestyle.

CHAPTER 12- FREE RADICALS AND ANTI-OXIDANTS

Free radicals are floating molecules that have an unpaired electron. Because the molecule is unpaired it floats freely, causing imbalance. It is very dangerous, hence the name radical. The molecule behaves like a radical as it seeks to steal electrons from other molecules in the body. When this process is happening at a high level, cells are unstable and some are destroyed. This process can result in premature aging and diseases.

Free radicals are the bad guys we hear about almost every day in health and wellness discussions, yet we cannot avoid them because they are the byproduct of normal metabolism. In addition, they have a positive side, as noted by Daniel Reid, "Free radicals play an important role in cellular defense by destroying bacteria and viruses, breaking down chemical pollutants, and neutralizing toxins."

The danger we hear about is because of an over-abundance of free radicals in our environment and food that overwhelm our body.

ANTI-OXIDANTS TO THE RESCUE

Because some free radicals are unavoidable, we must do something to minimize the adverse effects of these molecules, and that's where anti-oxidants come in handy.

ANTI-OXIDANTS

These are biochemical compounds that help to protect cells from the free radicals. There are numerous anti-oxidant vitamins and herbs that help to protect the body from free radicals.

Among the good antioxidants are vitamin A, C, E, fruits, and vegetables. Prunes are very high in anti-oxidants and blueberries are also good source.

CHAPTER 13 - STARVING CANCER

Cancer diagnosis is a scary thing to hear. The good news, however, is that cancer treatment has advanced over the years and today the range of available treatments are extensive ranging; from conventional, alternative, and complementary therapies. Cancer, like all diseases develops from something, and if we know what that "something is we can help prevent, treat, and possibly cure it.. Even after conventional or alternative treatment, we should try and eliminate the root cause. Research to find a cure for cancer has been in the forefront of medicine for decades and is still ongoing. Other research focused on causes and some have pinpointed several factors that are believed to contribute to cancer development.

These are:

• Diet: Numerous studies have shown that up to 70 percent of all cancers is dietary related. From consumption of red meat cured by nitrates and nitrites to an abundance of chemicals sprayed on the food we consume. Also a diet high in trans fats, processed foods, sugar, fried foods, and a lack of dietary fiber, fruits, and vegetables are all mentioned as dietary causes. Diets such as described above cause an acidic internal system that enhances cancer growth.

• Obesity: This is a huge factor in terms of causing cancer as well as many other chronic diseases.

• Environmental toxins of all kinds.

• Smoking and second-hand smoking.

• Stress and lack of exercise.

• Excessive alcohol consumption.

• Exposure to extreme sunlight without ultraviolet protection.

CANCER REDUCTION STRATEGIES

One of the best ways of staying cancer free is to help the body by focusing on the root causes mentioned on the prior page.

FOOD INTAKE

• Allow food to benefit your health rather than cause disease. All through history many studies have discussed the cancer fighting properties of several foods that are available to us.

• Eat a well-balanced diet with complex carbohydrates and a variety of fruits and vegetables:

✓ Tomatoes contain lycopene that fights free radicals.

✓ Cruciferous vegetables such as broccoli, kale, cabbage, turnips, and all dark green, leafy vegetables. They are packed with the cancer fighting properties of chlorophyll and magnesium, purported to cause cell death and prevent cancer development.

✓ Juicing a combination of green, leafy vegetables on a regular basis is excellent for overall health and for cancer fighting.

AVOID

• Obesity can trigger the growth of cancer. It is reported that an increase weight of 10 pounds increases cancer risk. Excess weight is a problem, so it makes sense to keep your weight within the normal zone. See the chapter on BMI to see the normal range.

• Sugar: All forms of sugar cause chronic inflammatory diseases because of the release of free radicals. Sugar may expedite the growth of cancer. Dr. Christine Horner states after extensive research, "Sugar is cancer's favorite food, the more we consume it the faster cancer grows." Scientific research is ongoing to validate this claim. It is safe to say, however, that excess sugar triggers obesity, and this in itself may contribute to cancer development. So it is best to avoid sugar. There are good sugar alternatives, like stevia on the market.[10]

• Fats from animals raised in confined operations described above, trans-fats, partially hydrogenated and hydrogenated fats — these are the bad fats that may cause heart disease, high cholesterol, stroke, and cancer.

• Xenoestrogens: These include any products that mimic estrogen such as BPA. This is the reason why there is such a fuss over BPA free water bottles and plastics.

• Soda and soft drinks. Most of these are loaded with sug-ar and produce the same health risks as described in the section on sugar above.

• Excessive alcohol consumption and smoking. These cause many health related problems.

• Pesticide-free foods. Some foods absorb pesticides more than others. The more common ones include strawberries, blueberries, and celery. It is recommended that we eat pesticide-free foods or organic where possible. If this is not possible there are food cleansing agents available or simply clean these fruits and vegetables with a combination of baking soda and vinegar.

• Environmental chemicals. There are many environmental chemicals. Certain chemicals in dry-cleaning as well as cleaning products are reported to cause cancer.

• Exposure to direct sun. Exposure to direct sun can cause skin cancer. Some skin cancers are very dangerous.

LIFESTYLE

Some lifestyle habits have been found to contribute to the development of cancer as noted in the prior section. Let's look at how we can change some of these areas.

• Avoid stress: Stress is difficult on the immune system. Extreme stress produces a breakdown of the immune system so the body is more vulnerable to develop cancer. Consider stress reduction initiatives that fit into your lifestyle. Some considerations include meditation, nature walks, listening to music, and aromatherapy.

• Exercise: Avoid a sedentary lifestyle. Exercise helps to reduce elevated insulin. Where there is insulin there is sugar. The goal is to reduce the amount of sugar floating in the blood where cancer cells can get the nourishment they need to grow. Some moderate exercise is helpful. You do not have to be a gym enthusiast, just engage in an activity that keeps the blood flowing,

• Smoking: Smoking causes many health related problems and is a contributing cause of many cancers. Avoid smoking as well as second-hand smoke.

• Sleep: Adequate sleep allows the body's cells to regenerate and improves overall performance.

CHAPTER 14 - STAYING OUT OF HOSPITALS

Hospital care in this country is based on an illness versus wellness paradigm. Other than natural services like childbirth or trauma care for accidents, the majority of services provided by hospitals are those designed to remedy complications from chronic diseases like high blood pressure, diabetes, high cholesterol, cancer, and inflammatory conditions. Millions of dollars are made by health care organizations that specialize in treating heart attacks caused from cardiovascular disease. Also, major centers are now built to treat cancer. The truth is that many of the conditions caused from chronic diseases can be prevented.

The hospital is not a place for healthy people. These huge structures can only stay open if you and I and others become ill. The number of wellness services that many hospitals offer is usually very small, and is the first area to be eliminated when there are budget cuts. The truth is that you do not want to be in a hospital bed unless it is an emergency situation that you have no control over. Many people die in hospitals, not from what they went there to be treated for, but from what the industry calls hospital, avoidable death caused by factors like wrong side surgery, falls, medical errors, medication mix ups, wrong procedures, and of course the most dangerous are the hospital acquired infections. According to the Center for Disease Control and Prevention (CDC), as many as 99,000 people in American hospitals die annually from infections acquired while in the hospital.

The more common of these are the Central line – associated blood stream infection, pneumonia, surgical site infection, C difficile, and Methicillin–Resistant Staphylococcus Aureaus (MRSA).[11]

The problem is so prevalent and dangerous that Medicare has reduced payments to hospitals if it is determined that the condition being treated and billed for was acquired while the patient was in the institution.

So why would a person want to be in the hospital if it could be prevented? If you are serious about living a healthy lifestyle and staying out of the hospital here are some things to consider.

CONSIDERATIONS FOR STAYING OUT OF HOSPITALS

One of the most important considerations for staying out of the hospital for chronic health conditions is to focus on prevention.

PREVENTIVE HEALTH

This area receives little focus yet is one of the most basic and foundational areas for wellness.

Think of your health care provider as a partner in wellness and not as a resource only for treating disease. Here are some suggested ways to partner with your health care provider:

• Have regularly scheduled annual physical checkups with your primary care physician. Most diseases, if caught early will have a better chance of being cured before they become chronic.

• There are certain tests that are recommended at various stages of life like mammography screening, prostate screening, colonoscopies, and pap smears. Get these tests when they are due.

• Know your numbers for cholesterol, blood pressure, blood sugar, weight, and BMI. Compare your ranges with normal ranges. Keep your test results somewhere with your health records so you can compare them each year. You can draw side-by-side comparisons by years so you can spot any changes. If any of your ranges are out of control, take action right away. Ask your practitioner how you can improve even without a lot of drugs.

• Maintain a healthy weight for your height. Calculate your own body mass index (BMI) The BMI is an index used to determine if a person is overweight. See the chapter on how to calculate your BMI.

• Avoid a sedentary lifestyle. Do some form of exercise. One size does not fit all, so not everyone needs to go to the gym. Some people enjoy walking, swimming, tennis, or a variety of other activities that get them moving. Find your own niche and do it.

• Avoid toxic build up. We cannot avoid toxins because they are all around us, but we can limit the amount we ingest by eating organic foods and cleaning fruits and vegetables properly before consuming them. A simple mixture of baking soda and vinegar will clean most fruits and vegetables. In addition, we can detoxify our bodies on a regular basis. Think about how often we change the oil in our car. Most dealers recommend at least every 2,000 miles because dirty oil will damage the engine and end up costing you more to fix. In the same vein we go through four seasons of eating different foods. We need to detoxify or clean out toxins from our bodies. Most practitioners recommend detoxifying at least quarterly, with the seasons.

• Get adequate sleep and avoid stress.

OUR DIET

Learn to eat for health rather than eating foods that can cause chronic health conditions.

• Avoid processed foods if you can. These may include white rice, pasta, crackers, and doughnuts because, in excess, they cause obesity, heart disease, impair the immune system, and expose the body to disease.

• Get adequate fiber in the food you eat. Fiber is a magic ingredient. In addition to helping you feel full, it helps to flush toxins out of the body.

• Keep your bowels open. Most diseases start with a clogged colon. According to Linda Berry, "Persons on the standard American diet hold eight meals of undigested food and waste material in the colon while persons on a high fiber diet hold only three."[12] Please note, when food stays in the colon for extended periods of time after the nutrients are extracted, it essentially rots and becomes a breeding ground for disease.[13]

• Avoid trans-fat and partially hydrogenated oils. These are normally found in potato chips, crackers, baked goods, and fried foods. These products may cause heart disease and bad health.

• Drink a lot of clean water each day. Six to eight glasses or more is good. If you are having a hard time consuming that much water you may try flavoring it with cucumber, mint, orange, or lemon. Also try sipping instead of drinking. Keep track of how much you drink each day and try to improve on it.

• Take vitamins that are not adequately present in foods, especially vitamin D3. In fact, ask your doctor to test the levels of vitamin D in your system at your next appointment.

• Stay away from junk foods like soda, potato chips, doughnuts, crackers, and other high glycemic index foods.

• Watch your sugar intake. Sugar is addictive and can harm your health.

LIFESTYLE

• Avoid alcohol, smoking, and exposure to direct sunlight.

• Have rest, relaxation, and fun in your life.

High blood pressure, heart disease, high cholesterol, cancer, diabetes, and pre-diabetes have at least one common causative element— obesity. According to Wendy Murphy of *USA Today Health Report*, "There is a direct relationship between increased weight and heart disease. Severely obese people are six times as likely to develop heart disease as those who are of average weight."[12]

She also reports that, "female hormones estrogen stimulate development of breast cancer, Overweight women produce 59 to 100 percent more estrogen than women of average weight."[13]

Therefore, if you are overweight and lose weight you could help decrease your chances of developing these chronic diseases. According to Dr. Lance Levy, "In understanding obesity, as little as a 10 percent reduction in body weight can reduce or eliminate an abnormal blood sugar by normalizing the action of insulin."[14]

Keeping a normal BMI is a key to avoiding many chronic health conditions. Review the considerations for staying out of hospitals and see which ones you can gradually incorporate into your lifestyle. If you do these basic foundational things you are on your way to helping yourself to stay out of hospitals.

ENDNOTES

1.   Freeman M and Junge, C. The Harvard Medical School guide to lowering your cholesterol. McGraw-Hill, two Penn Plaza, New York, 2005 : 118

2.   Herbert Victor and Subak –Sharpe, G. Total Nutrition. St Martin's Press, New York, 1994 ; 127, 46, 64

3.   Ibid

4.   Ibid

5.   Berry L. Internal cleansing .Three River Press, New York, 2002; 28 P44, 45 65.

6.   MacDonald M. Body Confidence. Harper Collins Publishing, New York, N.Y 2011; 36

7.   Levy L. Understanding Obesity the five medical causes. Firefly Books Ltd, Buffalo New York 2000 ; 72, 102

8.   Murphy W .Obesity, USA Today Health report: disease and disorders: Twenty-first century_books, 2012 ;18, 69, 74

9.   Bauer J et al. Food cures. Rodale Press, New York, 2007; 199, 133, 165

10.   Christine Horner. Waking the warrior Goddess. Read How you want LLC, 2009

11.   Article Source: http://EzineArticles.com/4514259

12.   Murphy W. Obesity, *USA Today* Health report: disease and disorders: Twenty-first century_books, 2012 ;18

13.   Ibid

14.   Levy L. Understanding Obesity the five medical causes. Firefly Books Ltd, Buffalo New York 2000; 102

ABOUT THE AUTHOR

Lena Dobbs-Johnson was trained as a registered nurse and spent over 35 years in health care leadership. Her most recent position was as a hospital executive. Prior to that, she held various senior-level positions in hospital settings. After leaving health care, Lena decided to pursue additional training and certification as a nutrition consultant and holistic health practitioner. Lena earned a Bachelor of Science degree in nursing from the University of Illinois at Chicago, a Master's degree in public administration from Roosevelt University in Chicago, a nutrition certification from Venice Nutrition, and a Holistic Science and Holistic Health Practitioner certificate from the Natural Healing College.

She is the recipient of numerous awards including the American College of Health Care Executive's Regents Award and the Chicago United Business Leader of Color.

Credentials
RN, BSN, MPA
Certified Nutrition consultant
Holistic Health Practitioner